POTTY TRAINING
in 3 days

A Step-By-Step Guide to Help Your Toddlers Go Free from Diapers

by Carol Moore

© Copyright 2020 by Carol Moore

All rights reserved.

This document is intended to provide correct and detailed information on the topic and problem. The publication is marketed with the understanding that the publisher does not make any accounts, officially approved services or otherwise suitable services. If legal or medical advice is required, an adult working in the field should be requested.

From a Theory Statement approved and ratified similarly by the American Bar Association Committee and the Publishers 'and Affiliates' Committee;

It is in no way permissible for any of this text to be copied, duplicated or distributed in any electronic or written media.

Recording of this publication is strictly forbidden, and the preservation of this text is not allowed until the publisher gives written permission.

The rights are all reserved.

The material presented herein is accurate and clear because the recipient's reader is alone and entirely responsible for the use or misuse of all of the rules, practices or instructions found therein in the case of inattention or otherwise. Under no circumstances should the publisher be found liable or guilty of reparations, damages or consequential compensation resulting from the herein contained material, directly or indirectly.

The copyrights not kept by the publisher are protected by the respective authors.

The material in this paper is only available for intelligence purposes and is thus basic. The delivery of the details is without consent or promise of any sort.

The logos used are without any permission, and the use of the mark is without the approval or support of the holders of the logo. Both trademarks and labels in this book belong to the owners and are not associated with this paper for clarifying purposes only.

Table of Contents

Introduction 8

Chapter One: 1,2,3… go! 10

    Is my baby ready to take the diaper off? 10

    Easy Transition 14

    Potty or Reducer? 21

    Essential Things 25

Chapter Two: Potty Training 33

    Potty Train your Child in 3 Days 33

    Day 1, Day 2 and Day 3 36

    Teaching to wash hands effectively 42

    Eating Habits and Diet 44

    Montessori Approach 46

Chapter Three: How to Fix Problems 50

    Potty Training Regression 50

    How to Manage Bedwetting 56

    The baby doesn't want to leave the diaper 65

Problems and Solutions 75
Conclusion **86**

Introduction

Tens of thousands of years ago there were no pre-birth courses or midwives who taught new parents the best way to put the diaper on their baby, indeed, the diaper didn't exist at all! Despite this, being able to "stem" the pee and poo of newborns has always been a problem that human beings have had to face since ancient times.

In warmer areas, children were left without clothes and mothers tried to promptly understand when their baby had to pee or poop while populations living in colder places had to cover their babies and ensure that they did not get dirty continually wearing heavy clothes.

In the most primitive civilizations, children wore animal skins which were then "stuffed" with moss and plants, materials which, once soiled, could easily be changed but which had poor absorbency and often caused skin problems.

In the Middle Ages, however, strips of linen were used as a diaper that were wrapped around the baby's pelvis and fixed with a safety pin.

In the following centuries, linen was replaced by cotton since it proved to be more robust and resistant to washing and with better heat dispersion, adapting more easily to the purpose. Cotton was the material of the "ciripà", a kind of absorbent triangle that takes its name from a population of Central America and their typical loincloths, which were wrapped around the baby and used as diapers.

Cotton was already an excellent material with a better absorbency than linen, but further progress was made in the mid 90's.

From the 1960s onwards, throughout Europe and North America, the first cellulose diapers were created together with a plastic pant that covered it. The latter, however, led to the creation of erythema in the child and therefore in the following years the quality of the diaper created only with cellulose was implemented. The diapers, however, were not disposable and were above all too bulky.

The greatest diffusion in North American and European markets occurred in 1961 thanks to Victor Mills, a chemical engineer, who for family needs, began working on this product in 1959 to launch it on the market years later.

Mills invented "Pampers" and he was the founder of the company that is still a leader in the sector. The spread of the "Diaper" product was rapid and is still considered a product that cannot be renounced.

Chapter One
1,2,3... go!

Is my baby ready to take the diaper off?

The baby seems ready and we would like to free ourselves forever from the burden of the diaper and move on to the potty, but a thousand doubts are gripping us: will it be the right time? Will my baby be ready for the big step? Will it be difficult for him / her?

It is by no means certain that the elimination of the diaper must necessarily be a tragedy. We often worry excessively and instead the business turns out to be simpler than expected.

Removing the diaper is an important step, which is reached on average around 2 years of age. But, as almost always in these cases, this is a rough indication: there are more precocious children, who take off their diapers at 18 months, and others a little lazier, who can reach two and a half or three years. Usually, at this age the child begins to understand the meaning of poop and pee and is able to communicate when she is about to do it. It is the right time to start. If you go far beyond this term, perhaps you should get a hand from the pediatrician. Actually, to understand when it is time to remove the diaper, there are some signals that the baby unknowingly sends and that can therefore encourage us to embark on this adventure.

When the child is ready for the potty

The first thing to note is if the baby shows discomfort from the wet diaper. It is now big enough for you to understand without misunderstanding. If as a baby she cried desperately, now she will tell you plainly that having a wet thing on her ass is really boring.

An element to consider is the fact that you will find the diaper dry or almost dry in the morning. In fact, if your child has not urinated at all or just a little during the night, she may be ready to potty. The same thing is true after the 2 or 3 hours during the afternoon nap.

Another sign could be that the child begins to put objects back in their place and the appearance of the symbolic play on this theme; for example, children may start putting their toys on the potty or be drawn to stories about this topic. Their minds are preparing to consider the potty as an appropriate place for their "products".

When your child goes from climbing stairs with both feet on the same step to going up stairs alternating feet (around 3 and a half years old). She will have greater self-confidence and greater balance.

Most importantly, your child needs to demonstrate an interest and a willingness to learn how to use the potty.

If your child is interested in keeping safe or clean and is curious about what you're doing when you visit the bathroom and wants to wear "big kid" underwear, your child is probably ready to get going.

You will encourage this curiosity by reading children's books and watching videos about using the potty and talking about it while you go about your everyday parenting.

The child becomes aware of her own body: she then begins to indicate the wet diaper with her finger and names body parts and body functions.

The child has achieved autonomy in dressing and undressing and taking off the diaper.

All these preparatory signals must attract the parents' consideration, but they must not rush them into imposing the autonomy of the potty.

When the child is not ready for the potty

The parent may misunderstand some signs that could make them think that the right time for the potty has come and, therefore, anticipate the request for its use but stop shortly after due to the child's refusal.

In fact, the child can correctly pronounce the word "pee" and "poop" but this does not mean that she is ready to use the potty because first, it is necessary to connect these words to the actual experience of relieving herself.

A child is not ready when she absolutely does not want to have her diaper removed, if she persistently opposes the potty or the toilet, or if she appears annoyed when a parent watches her before pooing. Since she experiences this moment with discomfort, it could mean that she does not recognize her own feces or pee as good parts of herself or she might be annoyed by the smell or texture of her own physiological products.

First of all, it is good to understand the causes of this attitude, this rejection is often more frequent in children who have a more difficult personality or in overly permissive parents. It is a good idea to suspend potty training for some time and then try again after a few weeks.

If the child goes away to defecate and does not seem willing to share this experience, it could mean that she is not ready for the "big step" yet but it is necessary to wait a little longer. If you try to potty train before this time, you're likely to run into trouble.

Another sign that a parent could get is the fact that the child starts standing in front of the potty or takes off her diaper and does her business on the floor, or when she starts to sit on the floor with the diaper all dirty and seems happy with the feeling she gets.

If she is still struggling to walk and run, she is probably not ready for potty training.

Easy Transition

Even though we can never quite know when our child is ready, potty training is like any other milestone, which is why we recommend getting prepared well in advance to avoid unnecessary stress and worry. Summer is perhaps the favorite season for parents to help children achieve this first great achievement of autonomy.

In addition to some practical measures, to accompany the children in this delicate phase, it is necessary to ensure that the context in which the path is undertaken is adequate to facilitate the achievement of the goal.

CALM PERIOD

Precisely because it is a delicate step, it is better to propose the transition in a moment of serenity for the child, avoiding unfavorable concomitances with other change events, and therefore stress (because children love routines and are reassured by them). Therefore, it is not advisable to start the phase of eliminating the diaper during a trip, close to the birth of a sibling or the beginning of kindergarten.

You can also wait for the summer: everything is easier in this period because the child is easier to dress, she can wear only a pair of panties at home, so you will avoid doing many washes of dirty clothes full of pee. In addition, the child spends more time with us in the summer, so you will be able to maintain a constant guideline throughout the day.

If you notice a discomfort in the child, rather than a desire to grow and a peaceful acceptance of change, it is better to suspend the process and postpone it to better times, this may not be the right time, but maybe after a month everything is easier.

ASK THE CHILD

In addition to preparing the bathroom with all the accessories you will need (at this time it is recommended to involve the child), you can go and buy the potty with her. When the time comes, you can ask her if she prefers to use the potty or use the toilet. If she replies that she would prefer the toilet, I recommend that you also buy the reducer and a toilet ladder so that the child can climb independently. Furthermore, this latter accessory will allow her to rest her feet giving her security.

NO PRESSURE TO THE CHILD

The transition is important, but it is better to avoid that all the attention of parents, grandparents, uncles and siblings is concentrated on the baby's pee and poop. Too much attention can be an excessive load of pressures and expectations for the little one, making her feel uncomfortable with the risk that she will withdraw into her comfort zone, refusing to commit to removing the diaper.

Never scold your baby if there are any minor inconveniences but remind her that you just need to call mom or dad and go to the bathroom. The inconveniences during this period will be more or less frequent, it does not matter. The important thing is to face them with the right spirit.

FAMILIARIZE WITH THE WATER

From when the baby turns 6 months or generally from when she learns to sit, you can decide to start familiarizing her with the toilet, using for example a potty or a reducer. Parents will have the task of recognizing certain signs (certain expressions, gestures, or particular crying and sequences) that the child is preparing to poop or pee, even before she begins to speak. When these signs appear, parents can get used to taking the child to the bathroom, making using the potty or the toilet a normal and daily gesture, even if not always productive.

Observing siblings or older friends in this sense can also help. You can introduce the potty as if it were a game from 18/20 months. Make her familiar with it for example by placing it in the bathroom, inviting your child to sit on it while, at the same time, you sit on the toilet.

READINGS ON THE TOPIC

Poop and pee are very dear to children, widely addressed by gender literature with stories and illustrated books that prepare the little ones to manage their needs independently. Reading books on the subject to children is certainly fun and can be useful in preparing them to do without a diaper.

Thanks to their help, you can face with more serenity all the various changes that the growth process brings with it as well as the abandonment of the pacifier, the arrival of a little brother, the beginning of kindergarten. These are all important steps for our children, which can sometimes scare them and at the same time leave their parents without the right words to say. So, reading a good book on the subject together can reassure and help exorcise worries.

Don't forget to place these books near the potty and the toilet so the child can pick them up and browse them even while doing her business. A useful way to relax.

When she goes to the bathroom, even if we don't sit on the toilet ourselves, we can sit next to her without rushing her and trying to relax her. We can tell her a story or read her a book.

CORRECT USE OF PHRASES

When it is time to go to the bathroom use affirmations with modality choice rather than questions. Even if she is not the one to tell you, you will entice her more without the use of direct questions such as: "Do you have to go to the bathroom?", "Do you have to pee?" to which you might say no. So, it's better to use a statement like "it's time to go to the bathroom" and then continue with a choice proposal based on the statement just made like "do you prefer to go with mom or dad?".

DON'T LOSE IT

Parents must avoid engaging in potty-training battles; these could disrupt the parent-child relationship and delay sphincter control; furthermore, there is a risk of chronic constipation and encopresis.

Accidents along the way are to be taken into account and can be tiring for parents to manage. So, you will need to have lots of patience and some practical help. You should equip yourself with waterproof protectors for mattresses, rugs and sofas and plenty of spare clothing (I'll talk about it later in the text).

Be constant and supported throughout the day in this choice (nursery, nanny, grandparents, etc.); the child must be able to live this phase serenely and not have different lines of conduct based on the people he is with. The rule must be one and only one: "you pee in the bathroom and don't wear a diaper".

NO PRIZES NOR PUNISHMENTS

Reproaches, punishments and blackmail, as in all things in life, have only counterproductive effects. So, try to respect the time of the child (it is useless to rage, if she really does not feel the urge to pee maybe she is not ready). Rewards are also to be avoided: the greatest satisfaction for the child will be to be able to poop without the use of a diaper, like older children. So, it will be fine to give her great verbal acknowledgement when she succeeds in this new achievement.

(Many parenting manuals recommend using rewards and prizes to potty train your child. However, you might ask yourselves how useful rewards and punishments are in general in the education of a child.

According to common opinion, the "good" child is the one who does not mess around, that respects the rules, that does not scream, that does not throw tantrums. A child that pleases the parent is effect of their will and she is not using her own self-determination.

Some believes that children's education manuals are very centered on the needs of the adult, on the automatic acceptance and preference for the rights of the parent, almost completely neglecting to take the child's needs, feelings and evolution seriously.

As with education in general, even in potty training, the reward that is given to the child for pooping under your command can be a trap that turns herself against the parents.

So, you need to reflect on why the child sits on the potty or does her homework alone and if this responds to her physiological need, to her internal motivation, to please the parent or just to have a game or something sweet.

Probably, with the rewards system, you would have hit our goal, there and then, that is to make our little one pee in the right place, but subsequently you would risk that she expects a reward every time just for having responded to a physiological need.

Then, tired of candy, should we offer something else to her, promising her something different every time?

No, on the contrary. If the little one does not want to sit on the potty, there is a reason and must be investigated. Promising a reward would only mean shifting the child's motivation from a response to a physiological need to a desire to please the parent. Or worse, denying the existence of her need such as that of peeing, in favor of an action carried out only to get something else from the outside.

The biggest motivation that pushes the child to be independent of the diaper is not so much the rewards, but rather the desire and the fact of becoming like mom or dad, older brother or cousin a couple of years older.

It is the desire to do it alone, which is why the parent should help the child to do it by herself without replacing her.

Potty or Reducer?

The potty is a known object that traditionally is used to remove the diaper, while the reducer is instead a new object to many people, an accessory that, as the name suggests, allows to reduce the seating space of the toilet making it more comfortable for children.

Unlike the potty, the reducer is inserted directly on the edge of the toilet so the child can sit in peace imitating adults but feeling completely at ease.

Suitable for any shape of toilet bowl, the reducer fits easily and it is comfortable both for the child who feels great and serene when using the toilet, and for parents who are not forced to carry pee and poo from the potty to the toilet.

Switching from the diaper to the reducer on the adults' toilet can be very convenient, more hygienic and also strategic to convince those children who really want to become and imitate adults. Furthermore, going directly to the toilet allows children not to make intermediate steps and not to have problems while traveling if there is no potty available around.

The reducer, unlike the potty, is linked to the bathroom, so it has a certain and clear location. The reducers on the market now meet every type of need: they are soft, colored and more or less compact.

Obviously, it is necessary that the toilet with reducer can be reached with a stool and that also everything necessary for washing is child-friendly and within their reach. Same goes for clothes: more than ever during this phase, clothing must be comfortable and easy. The jumpsuit is fine while the buttons and zips waste too much time.

For some, though, the potty is necessary since babies who want to poop and pee outside the diaper also want to see what they leave behind them! For children, in fact, the toilet can be too big and too deep (the "black hole") and does not allow them to see their businesses and where they end up.

The potty can be introduced into the home almost like a game, also due to its shapes that often recall cartoons, animals or toy cars. It is certainly the ideal solution to remove the diaper permanently in a playful way without creating anxiety in the child: the child can use it independently, without access problems, being at its height unlike the reducer.

The potty has also a small ergonomic seat, made to measure for young children and a structure with rounded edges slightly raised in the back, to rest their back comfortably, and in the front, especially to avoid splashes if this accessory is used by novice boys.

It is definitely recommended for those babies who are starting to can't stand the diaper or for those who are afraid of the toilet depth. The potty moves easily around the house; even if it is advisable to keep it fixed in the bathroom. This will give clear indications to children on the place used for poop and pee. There are also travel potties models: there are inflatable ones or cardboard ones that can be assembled and disassembled in no time.

If you are undecided whether to use one or another, you could propose both alternatives to understand together what facilitates the child. This would allow her to choose without pressure and become aware of her stimuli in freedom and comfort.

IF THE CHILD REFUSES TO USE BOTH

There are some children who, however, refuse to use both the toilet and the toilet. In these extreme cases, potty training can be started from another place. Close one eye on hygiene and try to make the first pee in the bidet, or in a basin or in a vase. If you have open space, you can propose to do it outside. Do not worry, this imaginative and atypical approach will last very little, and soon the children will be the first to want to go back to the bathroom voluntarily.

Little trick

One of the tricks that you can use to make your child go to the bathroom when she plays and do not want to stop is to ask her directly "do you want to go to the potty or the toilet?" instead of the usual "Do you have to pee?". You can continue to ask the question this way, even though the child always continues to choose the potty. In this way she feels that she is the one who decides, and as every parent of a 2/3 years-old child knows, the sense of independence and the desire to decide on their own is one of the most evident characteristics of this age.

POTTY

Pros

It is child friendly

The child often feels at ease because she can decide to sit alone

Helps the sense of independence

You can move it anywhere in the house

Cons

It must be emptied and cleaned after each use

It is not always available away from home, with friends, in a pizzeria, in a restaurant, etc.

At some point you have to agree to abandon it to start using the toilet

REDUCER

Pros

It is easily transportable by car and ready for use even outside home

You can leverage the child's instinct to imitate and show her how to do it

It is something that even adults use, and therefore the child can accept to use it more easily

You don't have to empty and clean it

Cons

Some children feel inhibited using it

Some children are afraid of falling into the toilet

Young children (1 year and a little over) need help climbing on the stool and sitting down on the toilet

Essential Things

One of the secrets of potty training is to make sure that you have all the necessary items and supplies before you begin.

Start with these and build up your child's interest in potty training.

This list of supplies will support you and your child to make this developmental milestone easier.

In the Bathroom

Potty Chair

Stand-alone potties are the right size for small learners and are available in a range of colors and familiar cartoon characters. A kid-sized potty is more straightforward to use and less daunting than a conventional toilet and can be moved around the house if necessary.

Seat Reducer

Smaller and cheaper than a potty chair, the seat reducer (or potty seat) sits on top of a conventional toilet and reduces it to a child-friendly level. Many of them have cheerful patterns and a padded pillow for added comfort. There are also folding versions that can be used both in public toilets and in emergency situations, but also for the home toilet. But beware that it is not always very stable and sometimes you have to keep the reducer still.

Stool

A small plastic or wooden stool can help your child get up and sit down on the toilet. It will also give your child a feeling of safety and security, so it will help you get her in the right place to use the toilet. A stool is also useful for lifting kids to the sink to wash their faces.

Toilet Paper / Flushable Wipes

Toilet paper is already standard in your loo but try to pick up a pack or two of flushable wipes. These are similar to baby wipes but disintegrate more quickly and are safer for plumbing. These wet wipes are softer than toilet papers, they are more familiar to your kids and make cleaning easier. Only make sure they are compatible with your plumbing.

Kid-Friendly Hand Soap

Potty training includes teaching good hygiene, so select a hand soap that facilitates post-potty hand washing. Try stocking up on foaming soap instead of a regular bar or liquid soap. Toddlers love bubbles, and there are simple, cheap recipes online to make your own once you've got a pump dispenser.

For Your Child

Choosing a potty is necessary, but so also is outfitting your little potty trainer for the job. From motivational undies to easy-to-remove pants, here are the things you need for your potty-training baby.

Awesome Undies

Cool potty-training pants and big-kid underwear can be a great motivator to help your child progress past diapers; anticipation is a crucial component of positive potty training. Imagine taking your potty trainer to the store with you to pick out her first pack of various colors, patterns, characters, and themes.

Easy On-And-Off Pants

During the first few days, weeks, and months of potty training, ditch the rompers, overalls, and button-up jeans for simple on-off pants and elastic waist shorts. Avoid using drawstrings or zippers to stop pants because they would need to be untied and unzipped. Your child will always have the impression that she needs to go, so you don't want to waste any time giving her complicated clothes; you want your child to be able to get the pants off in the shortest time possible, either by yourself or by your child. The goal is to teach your child to be self-sufficient enough to take off her pants and use the toilet, so pick a style that is easy enough for her to handle.

Training Underpants

Potty training pants in disposable and reusable/washable models are intended to make your child feel comfortable (unlike a diaper). That way, she knows when the potty is out, but the wetness is contained so that it doesn't soak into the clothing. For some families, training pants are a required intermediate phase in the potty-training process; for others, they may be a crutch that prolongs the transition from diapers to underwear.

Progress Chart

The use of a potty is a whole new habit for your kid, and it will help if she can see, chart, and remember her progress. There are a lot of beautiful charts that you can purchase on the web or print for free, but a simple hand-drawn grid decorated with your child should work. The goal is to help her — and you — note all the achievements that have been accomplished.

For Bedtime

Nighttime Potty-Training Underpants

Standard training pants are still not absorbent enough to accommodate an overnight period of 8 to 10 hours. Nighttime training underwear is more porous than their regular counterparts and is available in both disposable and reusable/washable models. They're a valuable transition item when your child works on daytime potty training as they can replace diapers.

Protective Mattress Cover

Sheets can be cleaned, and you can take care of an accident, but a soiled mattress is not an easy job to clean. Prevent this issue by purchasing a waterproof mattress cover: some are in plastic, and others have a light cotton top and a waterproof bottom sheet. Mattress covers may fit tightly over corners like a fitted sheet or wrap like a saddle around the middle of the mattress. Try investing in at least two covers to cope quickly with nighttime injuries.

Extra Sheets

Buy two or three sheets. Take a hint from seasoned parents and make a bed with at least two layers of sheets and a waterproof mattress cover. This way, if an incident happens in the middle of the night, you can easily take off the dirty sheet and the top layer of the protector and tuck your little one back into the bed with the dry bottom layer. Accidents happen, so you're going to save yourself from middle-of-the-night "fun."

Other Interesting Products That Will Help You

Pee Clock

There is a watch on the market that reminds the baby through lights and sounds when it is time to go pee. The music can be set in time intervals of 30, 60 or 90 minutes. It is very useful to prevent the first "accidents" that can happen to the baby who is trying to remove the diaper.

Mini Toilet

There are small toilets made especially for small children, complete with toilet paper and easy to clean, some also equipped with accompanying music.

Unique Potty-Only Activities

Whether your child has difficulty understanding the simple idea of going to the potty, is scared of the potty or is unable to spend enough time in the toilet, there is a wide range of potty training books, videos, and toys to make the potty cycle feel more familiar and less scary. Set down one or two books or toys that your kid would enjoy or find motivational books (which feature favorite characters in potty training) and dolls (which go potty or sing dumb songs about going number two). If you want to turn over your smartphone or tablet to your toilet trainer (which is not recommended as a daily practice), make sure to have a childproof cover and a screen protector that is waterproof like the new iPotty, a stand-alone potty with built-in iPad holder. However, be sure to follow the American Academy of Pediatrics' media guidelines, which do not prescribe a screen time for children under two and restrict the screen time to two hours a day for older children.

Stickers in the Toilet

It can help for boys to place funny stickers inside the toilet and encourage children to hit the stickers. Many parents want to start the boys in a sitting position, but if you want to encourage your son to urinate while standing, a specific toilet target may be a helpful device. These go inside the potty to ensure your little boy's target is the toilet bowl and not the walls. You may also select a cheaper option. A simple scrap of toilet paper may provide an amusing goal, when placed at the bottom of the potty. This is for boys who may need some motivation to aim.

Potty Training Rewards

New behaviors can be strengthened by encouraging accomplishments (although I personally disagree).

Start small with stickers, kid-safe sweets or all-natural fruit snacks, or some other little treat to make potty improvement. Brand-new potty trainers will need an incentive for every small victory (we're talking several times a day), but once your child has learned the basics, set long-term targets (five days without incidents, 25-time peering, etc.) to reward them with a prize.

Playing Area

Try to create a play area for children in the bathroom. Insert a small bookcase, a drawer with games, etc. so that even in the bathroom there will be a space dedicated to the child who will entertain herself while having fun. This will inevitably increase her affinity towards the area and can make her interested in the use of the toilet. This will help you enormously and with minimal effort.

Chapter Two

Potty Training

Potty Train your Child in 3 Days

You've finally decided that your child is ready to get out of diapers, CONGRATULATIONS!

The use of the toilet is a valuable skill that further strengthens your child's independence and increases her confidence. Toilet training aims to teach your children how to understand the pressure they feel in their bodies and when they need to use the toilet.

The most significant thing to remember is that potty training is a process, and your child will have many accidents, but stick to this approach, and your child will use the potty regularly in just three days.

Is Your Child Ready?

Before you decide to take a plunge and a potty train, you will familiarize your child with the use of the toilet. Let your child come to the bathroom with you and show her what "big boys" and girls are doing.

Most of the kids are excited to learn about the bathroom etiquette. Show them how to wash the toilet and how to wash their hands. Look for signs of preparation and anticipation, such as your child telling you when he or she needs to pee or poop, asking you to use a potty, feeling irritated with a dirty diaper.

Does your child seem ready to use a potty? The three-day strategy will work only if your child is on board.

Choose the Weekend

You'll need three days in a row when you're at home with your kids. For working parents, this approach works better on a weekend of three days or at a time when you can take a day off work to add to a daily Saturday / Sunday.

You'll be inside for most of the weekend, so it's important to brace yourself mentally to give a lot of time with your kids. Have fun with them. If you can't schedule out three days, on the last day, speak to your childcare provider about what you've been doing and ask them to continue the cycle.

Stock Up

When your child shows signs of preparation, take them to the store and pick up the underwear together. Buying underwear with their favorite characters is a fun way to get them excited about wearing big boys or big girl underwear.

Also, if you're going to spend a lot of time at home, you may want to think about some home improvements in advance. This could be art supplies, movies, sports, cooking, baking, or something else that keeps you and your child entertained.

Before the Long Weekend

Let your child know one week in advance that it's time to say "goodbye" to the diapers. Depending on what your family chooses, this could be a complete farewell or a partial farewell where diapers or pull-ups are used at nap and bedtime. When you start practicing, underwear must be worn at all times when your child is asleep.

If you're going to make a complete goodbye to the diapers, you should count the remaining diapers with your child and let them know that when they're gone, there's no more. It would help if you also made sure that only one diaper is left before bedtime the night before you start your toilet training.

Share the cycle with your spouse and other parents, such as nannies, babysitters, and family. Take turns (especially if there is an older brother) or stay together and support each other throughout the process.

It is vital that all adults are involved in the process and that the use of the toilet does not become something that can only be done with one person in the family. By sharing responsibility, your child learns that they need to use the bathroom with everyone, not just in certain circumstances or with particular adults.

Day 1, Day 2 and Day 3

DAY 1

Right when your child wakes, remove him or her from the diaper. On the first day, let the baby go around the house naked. This situation, which children generally love, will allow them to come into contact with their body and its needs.

You can opt to place a little potty in the living room for quick access. This is your choice, as some people might want to leave all the bathroom practices in the toilet. Give your child a huge cup of water, milk, or juice so that they have to pee regularly. Have a constant sippy cup within reach of your kids. Give your child a lot of liquid and look for signs that your child is about to pee or poop.

When you see the sign, take your child to the bathroom to use the toilet immediately. About every twenty minutes ask them if they prefer to do it in the potty or in the toilet (with the reducer). You might want to set an audible 20-minute timer so that your child knows that when the timer goes off, it's time to try using the toilet. Tell your child how to unfasten their pants, clean up after a toilet, and wash their hands. Clearly you will be the one to carry out these tasks, however listening to your words will slowly bring her closer to this ritual. In books or among some videos available online you will find songs and nursery rhymes to accompany this precious moment.

Before lunch, it's a good idea to go to the bathroom together. "I always have to pee before lunch and dinner. Let's do it together, then wash our hands and go eat." Encourage the child to sit on the potty while you are sitting on the toilet. after being in the bathroom, wash your hands and go eat.

After lunch, keep an eye on her to see if she struggles to evacuate. It is common for children to poop after lunch if they haven't done it in the morning.

Before napping or going to sleep, tell your child it is time to use the potty (avoid asking whether or not she wants to use it). Put on a diaper before falling asleep to avoid accidents. You can also choose to put her to bed without a diaper, it depends on what results you got in the morning. If you have put on a diaper, take it off when the baby wakes up.

If you wake the baby and the diaper or the bed are dry, praise her (if you have chosen to use the rewards technique reward her with a pebble or sticker). By the time there are three dry naps, the baby will have made great progress. After bed, take her to the bathroom and sit on the toilet while she is sitting on the potty. So, start introducing the habit: after bedtime you go to the bathroom.

Before dinner, follow the same procedure as for lunch.

Then follow the usual evening ritual, for example toothbrushing, pajamas, a little TV and reading a fairy tale. It is a moment of relaxation when you may want to pee. Keep the potty close at hand.

And when it's bedtime, tell the baby that all people sit on the potty or the toilet before going to bed to say goodnight to the last pee of the day. This also serves to establish a habit.

If your child does not desire to try, you could say that we're going to try "after you've finished playing with your toys," or, if your kids know numbers, you might say, "we're going to try when the clock says 10:00".

Try to use the bathroom at every changing phase of daily actions, for example after cleaning a toy/material, before a snack or lunch, and before and after a nap and bedtime. This will eventually become part of their daily routine.

Remember to use emotionally neutral behavioral observations about your child's progress. "You peed in the toilet, that's where the pee should be" or, "You peed on the floor? Let us clean it up together."

When the child is able to evacuate 10-12 times in the potty it means that she is becoming independent.

Hurray, she did it!

Celebrate the baby but don't overdo it or embarrass her.

You know your child best. Some children react well to an exciting celebration of achievement, while others are not at ease in this regard. If they react well to rewards, maybe your child would be excited about stickers or small treats (you can do a reward chart to encourage her potty training).

DAY 2

After the first day, you can use the diaper at night in order to avoid accidents.

The cycle for Day 2 and Day 3 is the same as Day 1. Some people stay inside for three days to solidify the process. On the second day, in fact, you can add another step: going outside for a walk with the child. Wait until your child has peed in the potty and then go out immediately. When leaving the house, make sure your child is wearing baggy pants with nothing underneath. They must not wear diapers or underwear. Your goal is to get out and back home without peeing on and without having to use the potty when you are out.

Think that in the East children are dressed in cotton shorts with a cut in the middle so that the little one can do his business anywhere in an agile way and be washed immediately, without the impediment of clothes. When you go outside, go to a park or do an activity nearby, and please remember to take a small portable potty with you in case your child fails to use the public toilet, as some children do. Expect accidents to happen. Only change the underwear as they happen, and don't make a big deal. Say to them, "We pee and poop in the potty."

DAY 3

The potty should be part of everyday life at this point. The day should go something like this:

- wake up, take off the diaper and potty within five minutes
- hand washing and breakfast
- clothes and teeth washing
- activities around the house or walk (after an hour and a half or two remind the child if she needs a potty)
- invitation to the potty before lunch and hand washing
- invitation to the potty before the afternoon nap. Put the diaper on before going to sleep. Sleep for about an hour
- wake up the baby and remove the diaper. Have her sit on the potty and leave her for three to four minutes (if she prefers you can stay with her in the bathroom to keep her company)
- afternoon ride. Potty before going out and after returning home
- dinner. Tell the child how proud of her you are
- after dinner, play quietly

- potty and baby bath
- fairy tales or TV, then potty before bed
- brush your teeth, last visit to the potty before bedtime. Put the diaper back on the night just before you say goodnight

If you don't get good results right away, wait about 6 to 8 weeks to try again. This is a technique that requires a lot of patience and time, but it will work

Potty Training Tips

Let your child use the toilet before leaving home and immediately after arriving at their destination.

Bring multiple changes of clothes and underwear before you leave.

Inform teachers, daycare providers, nannies, and babysitters of the signals from your child when he or she wants to use the potty and the words you use at home so that they can be familiar with your desires (i.e., pee, poop, toilet, potty, doo doo, BM as Bowel Movement, tinkle, etc.).

Going without a diaper is a new experience and some children can feel awkward or scary. Stay calm and encourage your child in this cycle. Research has shown that a negative response or punishment after an accident may contribute to a negative connection with pee or poo and may impede improvement.

Believe in the process. It's very tempting to get upset on Day 2 when your child has an accident, but if you do it on Day 3 and beyond, your child can show you that she knows what it means to be potty trained.

You can also use an "if, then" statement to your advantage. "If you're going potty, then you can play in the park." Choose a spot you know your child loves, like a playground or a ball pit. Think about all the fun things they like to do in there beforehand. Be very disciplined while there and tell them they have to potty before they play. (This is a good strategy if they have to go potty and they have to interrupt the play).

When they hesitate, tell them you're going home so they can't pee or poo on the playground equipment. Allow them to change their minds, but if they still refuse to go — and this is the most essential part — then go home.

Teaching to wash hands effectively

Washing your hands, even if before it was an important practice, now more than ever it has become a mandatory rule.

Children have the habit of touching many objects and then putting their hands in their mouths, but unfortunately the hands are an important vehicle for the transmission of germs and bacteria responsible for colds, flu, gastrointestinal diseases and more.

It is advisable to wash your hands before meals, after playing, after pooping or peeing, after sneezing or after returning home.

First of all, check that all the accessories that will be used for cleaning are present, such as non-aggressive hand soap suitable for children's skin, towel and a ladder to facilitate the baby in washing.

- - Start by washing the baby's hands with water that is not too cold or hot
- - Put the soap on the baby's hands (preferably liquid because the classic soap could retain germs) and begin to lather the back of the hand, fingers and nails for at least 30 seconds (there are those who even reach 60 seconds), singing a song to make the moment pass a little more playful and cheerful
- - rinse hands thoroughly with running water to remove any trace of soap that may be left under the nails
- - remember not to touch the tap with your hands (especially if you are in a public bathroom) and dry your baby's hands with a clean towel or an air dryer

In short, washing hands can be considered a kind of do-it-yourself vaccine, simple, cheap and without side effects.

Eating Habits and Diet

Give your child high fiber foods, such as fruit and vegetables, wheat bread, and high fiber cereals, to obtain the right stool consistency. It is common for children to be "picky" eaters during the toddler era.

It is important to never miss fruit and vegetables from your table and to have a diet as varied as possible. If children are exposed from early childhood to a wide variety of foods and flavors, the more likely they are to enjoy them.

Here are some ideas that could benefit you:

If your child doesn't like food, give small portions and praise to your child for trying one or two bites.

Restrict milk to 16 ounces of low-fat milk and, if constipated, restrict all dairy products.

Provide fresh fruit instead of sweets and snacks.

Actually, children are able to regulate themselves by taking the amount of food they need, so you shouldn't force them or scold them if they don't want to eat. The energy requirement varies from child to child, based on the pace of growth, weight and activity she does, so it is good not to get anxious about this subject.

Even at this stage, your child's diet must be as varied as possible, it is better to limit the amount of sugar and salt and favor simple cooking, without too much fat. The best dressing is extra virgin olive oil used raw. Be careful not to use food as a reward or consolation and teach your children to sit at the table and avoid letting them eat in front of the TV or while playing.

Better to prefer steam cooking, excellent for vegetables and fish, because it reduces nutritional losses, or in the oven, which allows you to cook without adding fat. Even pressure cooking, speeding up preparation times, reduces the dispersion of nutrients. And if the vegetables are boiled, keep in mind that salts and vitamins pass into the cooking water, which can be reused to prepare soups or cook pasta.

It would also be useful to eliminate (or at least limit) the following foods from the diet of children:

- - French fries, which contain a carcinogen that forms during cooking
- - gummy candies, which are full of sugars, dyes and jelly, toxic substances
- - fruit juices, a product that contains many added sugars (it would be better to choose a 100% fruit product)
- - carbonated and sugary drinks, for the reasons mentioned above.

Montessori Approach

I would like to refer to one of the fundamental figure of Italian and world pedagogist of the twentieth century because I think she did an amazing job on children, Maria Montessori. Mother of Scientific Pedagogy, she was also the creator of the "Children's Houses" and had exported her method all over the world.

She was also an active supporter of the battles for women's emancipation, for the recognition of the rights of people with deficits, the poor and the exploited.

A multifaceted woman that dedicated herself to study and research for the improvement of society through education, with the hope of being able to build, through it, a world of peace.

To help the baby to eliminate the diaper, first of all, ask yourself if she wants to remove it and how you can help her in this achievement. This is because in the Montessori philosophy the importance of the child and her self-determination is always placed at the center.

Referring back to the basic principles of Maria Montessori's thought, we can say that it will be fundamental:

Follow the child, her speed and her needs;

Love the child, show affection, offer strong emotional support;

Stimulate and encourage her to search for independence;

Create a suitable prepared environment.

If the child does not progress, going back is absolutely not a defeat. The child is likely to be focusing on improving some other skill.

The child will understand for herself when the right time has come and will let us understand. We must favor the child and not judge her. This will increase self-esteem and self-confidence and then face the surrounding world.

Here are some Montessori tips for getting rid of the diaper

- take advantage of the *right* moment when the child is ready and not according to the season. It is important not to postpone that moment

- always change the diaper in the bathroom since the child will identify this place with her physical needs

- change the diaper in an upright position, this is because the child will associate the position with taking off her panties, as well as the fact that it is much more comfortable for her (make sure the baby can support herself on her legs).

- go to the bathroom with her or take her to the bathroom if she wishes

Going to the bathroom and using the toilet must become a natural thing and must not be a mysterious circumstance. She will observe through the example of his parents. Feeling close to someone will somewhat eliminate the stress when you have to do something for the first few times.

It is advisable to avoid sitting on the toilet as an obligation even though many parents leave their children sitting as a punishment until they do their business. On the contrary, Montessori recommends waiting for a warning gesture that indicates that they want to go to the bathroom.

— create a space for the baby in the bathroom

as I said before, it is important to create a suitable bathroom area for the child in which she can feel comfortable. You can add the potty, children's books that she can browse freely.

Montessori explains that to take advantage of their autonomy, it is important that children do not feel that they have to depend on others to solve their problem. If you have a potty, a stepladder to use the toilet, or a reducer, it's important that they find them within easy reach. When they understand that they want to and that they can go there alone, it will be easier for them to do so, if everything is ready

— avoid rewards technique

The child is reaching part of her natural development and this is not a special action, a talent or a mission that deserves to be rewarded

- do not scold her or make negative comments

This is absolutely to be avoided. I will never repeat this concept enough: with children it pays to be patient, to be loving and not to be angry at their apparent clumsiness. The motivation towards success must prevail in this path. Try not to give importance to the event, teaching it without taking it back and without causing further agitation in them. Children need to understand that this is a normal growth process and, when they feel wet, they will naturally predispose to use the potty.

If we set out to take the path of removing the diaper, it is useless for us to take it as a commitment with an exact deadline. We allow children to go at their own speed.

Chapter Three
How to Fix Problems

Potty Training Regression

The development of children, in every sphere of life, never follows a straight line, never always and only goes forward, but it may happen that for a certain period it stops or that some steps can be taken backwards.

This also happens with regard to the acquisition of sphincter skills: suddenly, after months and months from having eliminated the diaper, when the control of one's own needs had become the normality for the child, accidents return frequent and parents are understandably alarmed.

To distinguish whether it is a simple accident or a small phase of regression, it is first of all good to understand if the child had already manifested in some way that she had to go to the bathroom and, for a matter of timing, she was unable to hold it or if the "accident" (or more than one) occurred without any previous signal.

In the first case it can happen even if you are not going through a regressive phase, simply due to the fact that children have times and rhythms that do not always coincide with those of adults; in the second case, especially in the presence of repeated accidents, one could speak of regression.

But don't worry about that. Regression can be corrected. It's just going to require some retraining, patience, and listening to get back on track.

What Can Parents Do to Help?

Even though your child seems to have mastered going to the potty, a new situation can throw them away. Their attention and energy are on the new thing, not on staying dry and finding a bathroom. They may also lose interest temporarily once they have mastered the potty, especially if there was a lot of fanfare and attention to toilet training. In reality, so-called regression is a fairly common phenomenon. In fact, the development of the child is not linear and always ordered.

Regression can sometimes happen to older children, too. Changing schools or bully can trigger a setback. Children who are mentally and emotionally overwhelmed may ignore the signal of their body to head to the bathroom.

Accidents can happen when a child is under stress. Anything new or different can also cause extreme stress for children.

These situations may lead to a regression: a new sibling, new school, a different kindergarten, a new parent routine, social changes in the family, etc.

This stress can be minor and temporary, just like when your child is exhausted or distracted by playing.

Here are some of my advice to help your children:

STAY CALM

Even though you're frustrated, remember that a period of regression can be normal. It could happen for several reasons, but it can be fixed.

DON'T PUNISH

Experts say that punishing your child for bed-wetting or any accident is only a backfire. Bedwetting, in particular, is not under your child's control. And punishing accidents makes it more likely that your child will try to avoid punishment by hiding or trying not to poop or pee at all, leading to constipation and even more accidents.

CONTROL

Check the baby's pee as much as possible by making her go to the bathroom at set times such as when she wakes up, after breakfast, before going out, before going to sleep.

OFFER POSITIVE REINFORCEMENT

Clean up accidents and move on. Give your child the attention they want to take to other good habits: at preschool, at the table, washing their hands, etc.

It feels great for any of us to hear that we're doing the right thing. Give a lot of hugs, kisses, and cuddling. A sticker chart or a treat after a successful toilet stop works well for some children as well.

FIND OUT WHY

Accidents in older children are often linked to a lack of control over the child's environment. Try to get into their heads and find out what's going on. Understanding the cause can help you figure out the solution. Talk it through and open up the issue.

SYMPATHIZE

You should recognize that you know it's hard to keep up with everything that's going on in your child's life. You can use a childhood story about a time when you regressed and tell them that it can be normal.

REINFORCE TRAINING

Remember, what you did before initially worked. You can reinforce that with a set time to sit on the potty. It may be before nap time or after the bath or mealtime. Make it part of your routine. Endeavor not to make a big deal about using the toilet and don't force the issue, add it to your child's day.

MAKE EXPECTATIONS CLEAR

Make your child know that you expect them to return to the potty and to have clean undies. Let them know that you know they can do this.

DON'T MAKE COMPARISONS

Avoid making comparisons with other babies by saying for example: "Look, Tommy has already taken off his diaper! What are you waiting for?".

Don't compare your daughter to her brother, her little cousin, her classmates. And don't allow it to others either. Each child is a unique, unrepeatable person. This will lead to negative effects on both the self-esteem and the serenity of the child, who instead needs to compare only to herself to be more aware of her own potential and progress.

If the child is confronted with a positive thing, she may feel the need to always be the best for fear of disappointing. Conversely, if compared to a negative thing, she will get frustrated and will end up hating the person she was associated with.

This tendency to always be under judgment feeds the fear, anxiety and shame of children, emotions that accompany their lives and that break down their self-confidence.

SEE YOUR DOCTOR

Give your pediatrician details of the regression. You want to prevent the possibility of infection and make sure you're on the right track.

Language

Cute and technical language are both fine.

During potty training sessions, parents often wonder what kind of terms they should use with children. Is language such as "bowel movements" or "urine" proper, or should parents use more informal terms such as poop and pee?

Whether to use clinically correct terms for body parts or digestive waste, is a highly personal decision and often based on one's family history, people whose parents used "pee" and "poop" are likely to use these terms with their children.

Nothing is wrong with either style. You're not going to do any injustice or harming your child by using childish words to describe these things. She is a child, after all, and unless you're planning to hide her away, she will finally learn both the correct words and some slang that will make you absolutely cringe.

I think it is not the use of words but most of all the embarrassment that a parent makes the child feel about his or her private parts or about having to evacuate that can cause the child to become inhibited.

Potty Language Should Not Be a Language of Shame

As I said before, as a parent, you shouldn't associate nudity or the baby's private parts with something embarrassing or ashaming. This could cause unjustified embarrassment in the child who will be reluctant to show her genitals to pee or poop, thus delaying her adaptation to using the potty.

My dispassionate advice is to use any term you want without showing bad emotions such as anger, anxiety, resentment etc.

How to Manage Bedwetting

All children get the bed wet sooner or later during the night. But how can this problem be solved?

It can take some time for your baby to learn to stay dry all night. The process that leads to knowing how to control the bladder usually takes place around the age of 3/4, but up to the age of 5, bedwetting should not be considered a concern.

However, when it happens it is stressful for the child and frustrating for the parents. However, the family can intervene with some precautions to try to avoid (or at least contain) the phenomenon. The important thing is to always remember that you should not make the child feel guilty, but you must try to reassure her and make her feel more confident, so that she will undertake not to wet the bed.

A contributing factor to bedwetting is the fact that the child has a deeper sleep than adults. This means that, while the adult that has a full bladder, still feels the urge to urinate and wakes up to go to the bathroom, the child sleeps in such a deep sleep that she does not feel this stimulus and therefore gets wet. In addition, the baby's tissues retain more fluids than adults and are able to absorb a fair amount of water which then flows into the bladder.

Instead, psychological factors alone can facilitate its occurrence but are not the cause of bedwetting. Problems at school, arguments between parents, a move, the birth of a baby brother are stressful events that can give rise to various psychosomatic disorders: some children may express their discomfort with recurrent abdominal pain, others with vomiting and still others with enuresis.

Here are some of the tips I can give you if this problem happens.

− First of all, it is important to establish a dialogue with the child and possibly you can talk to her about your experience when you were little. Communication with the child is always fundamental and it is right not to forget the episode. By doing so, the child feels and is sure that the problem is resolved at some point. You have stopped having it in bed after all. Also, your child will feel less embarrassed by talking about it.

Always be comprehensive and be a reassuring figure to her as much as possible.

You can also explain to her the technical reasons that led to bed wetting. Obviously, providing more understanding on this subject will help.

- Another reason could be the fact that she drinks a lot before bedtime and therefore, a solution, to limit drinks the two hours before sleep (especially liquids that promote diuresis). Although it cannot be considered a definitive solution and although it is not always practicable, limiting the consumption of drinks, especially carbonated, in the hours preceding the moment of sleep, can help to contain the problem. It is important, however, that the child drinks enough and regularly throughout the day.

- You can train her bladder to make it larger. In fact, among the possible causes of enuresis, there is that of having a low capacity of containment of the bladder which tends to empty as soon as it reaches the maximum filling.

In these cases, the child can get used to 'hold' the pee for a longer period of time during the day, extending the interval between two successive excretions, so that even at night the holding period can increase.

- The use of absorbent panties is particularly useful since, on the one hand it allows the child to have a peaceful sleep and, on the other hand reduces the stress of parents who are not forced to wash sheets and pajamas every morning.

Remember always to empower the child without having to resort to useless scolding and above all without making her feel ashamed, getting help in cleaning and changing sheets. This helps the child to feel she can contribute positively.

- Even if you have the urge to wake her up in the middle of the night to make her pee, this is not recommended. However, some parents, before going to sleep around 23-24, wake up the child (from 5 or 6 years old) and take them to the bathroom to pee.

Despite the child must be able to enjoy adequate quantity and quality of sleep, remind her to always go to the bathroom before going to bed.

- You can also create a calendar with dry nights and wet nights and stick stickers on it and remember to praise her if she left the bed dry.

Alarm systems are also used, especially in the Nordic countries, to warn the baby when she is getting wet. It consists of two parts, an extremely sensitive control unit that uses the most advanced electronic techniques, and a lightweight and comfortable detector pad that is placed on the mattress cover and the sheets, then covered with a smaller sheet. As soon as the first drops of urine touch the pad, the alarm emits a loud sound that wakes the child. It is a system that works quite well, but which in many countries is reserved for children who do not respond to other treatments because it associates enuresis with a nuisance stimulus, sometimes interpreted as a bit punitive. In fact, it is usually the last resort.

Do not think about reusing diapers anymore.

How to eliminate stains and odors

First of all, know that there is a way to prevent your baby from dirtying frequently. In fact, there are absorbent sleepers on the market that you will have to place practically everywhere (in the bed, on the sofa, in the car) and always carry some with you until your child is independent. There are also washable ones, cheaper and certainly less polluting in the long run.

This will allow you not to lose our temper if an "accident" occurs and you will be able to continue this transition period in the most rational way possible.

In addition to removing urine stains and related halos on clothes, mattresses and perhaps the car upholstery, remember that you will also need to eliminate the persistent stench.

Here is the procedure to remove stains with the help of household products:

1. Dilute some hand laundry detergent in cold water and blot stains. You can pour the resulting solution into a spray bottle for convenience.

2. Mix water and white vinegar in equal proportions. Blot or steam the area to be treated.

3. If you have forgotten or did not have time to treat the stain before and it is already dry, sprinkle it with baking soda and leave it on for the whole night; allow at least 12 hours to pass, then remove the grains with a brush and proceed with the normal washing.

4. If you are facing a stain that does not want to go away, you can combine the mixture of water and white vinegar with baking soda; first proceed with the powder and then with the liquid solution, let the mixture act and remove it only when it is completely dry.

Borax may be possibly used for this purpose. It is produced by the reaction between boric acid and soda. Before using it, clean the area with a mild stain remover. Immediately after, sprinkle some borax on the patch and stick some paper towels well. After about half a day, remove the borax residue and move on to washing.

MATTRESS

The most important thing to do in case the mattress is wet with pee is to absorb the stain as much as possible. If the stain is fresh on a material that cannot be submerged in water, the very first thing to do is to dab the stain with dry cotton rags and press it to remove as much liquid as possible. The area must be buffered and not rubbed, in order to prevent the urine from penetrating even deeper or worse still from spreading. Only then can you proceed to treat the stain with the methods described above.

When the rags no longer get wet from the stain contact, we can begin to disinfect the area with a solution made up half of hydrogen peroxide and half of white vinegar. In this way we obtain a very powerful disinfectant which also has the advantage of deodorizing. The solution should be dabbed on the stain with other clean cotton rags until you no longer smell the stench.

If, on the other hand, the fabric can be removed and washed, you can only do the first step indicated and then you can throw everything in the washing machine.

While if the pee is already dry or the stain is already dry, proceed directly with the bicarbonate mix and a mixture of water and vinegar. At the end of this operation, make sure that the mattress is dry. If necessary, use a hair dryer or fan.

If the yellow stain is present, when the disinfection is finished, it must be removed with only hydrogen peroxide that is rubbed with a white patch and then it can be left to dry directly on the fabric, perhaps with the help of a low temperature hairdryer to speed up the operation increase the whitening effect of hydrogen peroxide.

CARPETS

Not much can be done on carpets, but you can still give it a try in the laundry.

If the stain has been done recently, however, you can proceed in this way:

Sprinkle the stained area with baking soda or corn starch until it is completely covered. Leave it there for as long as possible (24 hours would be perfect) and then scrub with a soft bristled brush. You will understand if the process has been successful because grains will form which must then be removed.

However, if the damage seems particularly serious, mix the baking soda (or corn starch) with cold water and rub it on the stain trying to avoid damaging the texture of the carpet.

The method just described is also valid for car interiors or any other type of upholstery, as well as for the pee of any pets.

CLOTHES

Again, if the stain is recent, the first thing to do is to dab to remove most of the urine.

When it comes to clothes, it will be necessary to use something that disinfects and at the same time has the ability to deodorize. Create a mixture of 12vol peroxide and white vinegar in equal parts and tap the stain until it disappears. But be careful not to overdo it: the result could be a nice yellow spot.

If this happens accidentally, add a whitening product to your usual detergent in the washing machine. Try not to use the dryer because the heat would end up fixing the stain even more.

For light-colored fabrics such as white ones, it is better to opt for a pre-wash with hydrogen peroxide: not only is it stain-remover but it is also a disinfectant. Just use it in combination with water (in a proportion of 1/6, so for a tablespoon of hydrogen peroxide we will use 6 of water). In the absence of hydrogen peroxide, it is also fine to use vinegar, in slightly higher proportions.

Training panties - a great help

They are simply a wonderful invention for parents who are having problems with potty training. With them you can say goodbye to diaper rash, eczema, irritation and all the problems from transition to the toilet in a natural way.

One type of panty resembles the diaper. This model is made of a special sponge that absorbs just enough so as not to get the legs and feet of babies wet and prevent them from feeling discomfort (the absorbency depends on the amount of urine) and a waterproof outer layer. They are perfect when you are away from home and you are not sure to get to the toilet on time, such as during car trips but also during naps.

They can be removed and put back on. These panties leave the baby feeling wet to let her know that it would be better to go to the bathroom just after the stimulus.

There are also ecological models with the internal absorbent layer and the one in contact with the skin made of breathable cotton and corn starch, while the elastic containment bands and adhesive parts are made of recyclable plastic. Definitely a good way to reduce pollution.

The other model is less bulky than the first, has less absorption capacity and has a non-waterproof outer layer. This special panty can be suitable for those children who want to tell parents when to go to the bathroom but who involuntarily lose a few drops of pee (not suitable for heavy losses). They are very comfortable to take off and put back on and allow the child ample freedom of movement.

The baby doesn't want to leave the diaper

Taking off the diaper is an achievement that has different times and ways.

For most children this happens quite naturally, almost abruptly. Parents ask her to say when she needs to pee, they invite her to use the potty or the toilet directly with the reducer and it may take a couple of days to do so, if the child is ready.

For other children the path is more difficult. There is a sort of affection to the diaper, which gives security.

It can be a ploy to take off her diaper and put her panties on. The child, pissing herself off, will perceive a sense of annoyance so next time she may think about it before doing it or warn her parents.

But each child is unique. Precisely for this reason, it may happen that your little one will hold his pee for 24 hours, consciously, in order not to use the potty.

It can also happen to put her on the potty, to spend a lot of time humming, playing and chatting without getting anywhere.

When she can no longer hold her pee, she will invoke the diaper. If she is put on the toilet, she won't do it anyway. Small gimmicks such as tickling or running water will not stimulate urination.

If you are stubborn and don't allow the baby to use the diaper, she will eventually pee herself off, crying desperately.

Very often, the refusal of the potty is due to trauma. Specifically, something scared the baby, giving her insecurity the first few times when she took off the diaper.

It takes very little to traumatize the child. She may, in fact, have heard a door slam while on the potty, a reprimand if she wet her panties, etc.

Precisely for this reason, the best thing to do is to have a lot of patience. When the child is on the potty, you have to create a relaxed environment and have to be careful of noises, moderating the tone of voice.

Then, avoid insisting and try to converse with her. Don't worry too much if a lot of time goes by without the baby peeing.

Surely, in this delicate phase the child should not be reproached when she gets dirty, otherwise she will close herself off even more and everything will become difficult. Rather, let's praise her when she can understand the urge and go to the bathroom, encourage her with every little step forward.

That said, it is obviously normal to be 'forced' to give a diaper at some point, otherwise the kidneys and bladder would be put to the test.

Problems with poop

Every mother knows their babies well and will be able to recognize when they are forcing themselves in wanting to eliminate the diaper early. You must always take into account the progress of the child, but at the same time, do not insist too much and do not have too many expectations, trying to see how things are progressing as you go along.

It can happen that the child is in difficulty and rejects the urge to poo, or because they get dirty without a diaper or because, for example, they are forced to stop playing to reach the potty. In these cases, a constipation problem can occur. It takes a lot of calm and tolerance, even here it is essential not to put pressure on the child, otherwise you risk doing worse. You can wait up to 2/3 days of abstinence, then it will be necessary to stimulate the child with a glycerin suppository: at that point the advice is to put her on the potty, keep her company by playing or reading a story until she has done the poo.

Some babies may develop a form of stool retention and ask to use the diaper again. However, if they use it as if it were a potty, for example by hiding while they poop and using it only when they poop, it is good to give it to them. They are still doing the correct "gesture" and will soon be ready to sit on the potty.

For the child, feces represent a part of himself that often struggles to let go.

A technique that can be used if you see the child in difficulty with their poop is to create a moment of play, for example by proposing suitable readings for their age, leaving the children in their intimacy and showing you available only if they request it.

Another strategy is to participate with them in the joy of what they have produced, to let go of the feces and greet them. This is a small action that gives peace of mind to the child who peacefully detaches herself from her "product" and which is taken into consideration by the parent.

These are some hygiene rules that might help:

- get your child used to going to the bathroom at the same time every day;
- make her sit on the potty, or on the toilet with the help of a reducer and a stool, so that her feet are well supported and assume the correct position a little squatting;
- if, with the first attempts to remove the diaper, you understand that the child is reluctant to evacuate, it is better to take a step back and put the diaper back on for a few more weeks;
- do not keep the baby sitting on the toilet or potty for too long: if after about ten minutes she does not evacuate, better try again after a few hours.

In addition, you can tell the child who is trying to poop, making some effort: "dear, you are feeling this way because it is your poop that is asking you to let it out. Let it out. Only you can help it with that."

So, let's give the child power over their own bodies. Obviously, this is a different approach to manipulation or distraction to doing something only to please parents or make them happy.

Also try to dampen the child's performance anxiety, avoiding calling grandmothers, aunts and various relatives to ask if the child has pooped. Thus, monopolizing attention will make things more difficult and hinder them.

I advise you to buy low-cost underwear so as to be more relaxed if you have to throw some of them away.

To improve the child's defecation, avoid external intrusive maneuvers such as microenemas or external stimulations, unless they are advised by the pediatrician and always follow his help. This will cause the child to lose body awareness and mastery will worsen. The more you make your baby poop artificially, the harder it is for her to become familiar with that mechanism.

Sometimes a child may feel sorry for their poop going down the pipe. In fact, at the beginning it is good to use the potty so that the child looks at her products and can reassure herself. You can explain the process that happens to poop after it has ended up in the sewers. For example, you can tell her that through a long journey it reaches the sea to feed the fish, or that it is transported and used to fertilize the surrounding fields and trees. Probably with these explanations she will better deal with the "loss".

Hard Stools

We talk about constipation when the feces are hard and appear as pebbles (goat feces). The child may feel a lot of discomfort or pain during evacuation and the stools may show traces of blood due to the rupture of blood vessels in the anal region during their passage.

To identify constipation in children you also observe that there is no bowel movement for 2 or 3 days longer than usual, bowel movements are hard or painful, stools are large and can clog the toilet, or, as we said before, there are drops of blood on the external stool.

The fear of seeing these episodes repeat themselves in the bathroom pushes children to try to avoid defecating at all costs. The more they hold it, the more the feces dehydrate until they become real stones.

The presence of occasional constipation should not cause concern, but it is important to consult the pediatrician when the situation tends to become chronic and if bowel movements with the presence of blood tend to be frequent.

A temporary intestinal obstruction can result from a minor trauma that caused the baby to poop in a somewhat painful way. That's why she is scared and may hold back from doing it.

One thing your pediatrician might recommend is to give your child special syrups to make their stools softer and more voluminous.

Other things that can help the transit of feces are to increase the intake of fiber, therefore fruit and vegetables. Since this can also happen due to not drinking enough, get your child used to drinking more throughout the day. Avoid packaged foods or foods that have undergone a long process of transformation. You can add a glass of warm water with lemon to your child's diet and let her drink it every morning.

Prevent your child from having a too sedentary life and make her do physical activity. Just take it to the park and let her run for hours. The movement, in fact, facilitates intestinal evacuation.

Problems with pee

Keeping the pee and poo, which the child reaches around 2/3 years, represents a very important evolutionary stage like weaning. The child learns control over herself and begins to listen to what she needs without the parent telling her. Being a very delicate phase, it should be faced by the parent with patience and serenity. The fact that the child holds on to pee or poop could be seen as holding back emotions and the reason should be investigated.

Criticizing her, judging her and making her feel "dirty" is wrong and absolutely to be avoided. The baby will get frustrated, so you better do not pile it on. Do not associate the idea of urination with something bad, to be abhorred. The result will be that "if it is a dirty thing it will be better to hold it". It would be advisable to change your mind and make the child understand that peeing and pooping are not negative events, but they are nice things to do because they free themselves and feel better. You can ask the baby just as she evacuates if she feels better or worse. Surely the parent's behavior is not deceptive but pointing out your child as a "slob" is to be avoided.

Always remember to praise the baby who goes to the bathroom, singing her funny songs that she will associate with a happy and carefree moment.

Remember not to reward or punish preschool children, especially on things that affect the child's body such as food and toileting. This is normal and physiological. If instead it becomes something that the child does to please the parents, remember that then she can use the same method with you: she may not go to the bathroom so the parents "do not win" or to keep attention on her. This, from a physiological fact, passes to the relational field. Instead, you can empower the child by telling her that pee and poop are her stuff and they, if she wants, can be managed together with the parent.

Right after pooping or peeing, instead of telling her she was good, say "Wow! You saw how better it feels! Even mom feels a lot better when she does it".

Always rely on your pediatrician especially if you think the problem comes from a more serious cause (such as a urinary tract infection) and try to detect when the disorder has emerged. So, you will understand if there was a trigger or not.

Fear of the toilet or washing hands

Fear of getting dirty is common in children and can represent an excessive attempt to control one's body. This excessive control can arise from difficult emotional management. An emotional condition that is difficult to control may be present in the child, which is expressed in self-control behaviors from which the excessive fear of getting dirty arises.

It is usually an anxiety that disappears naturally with the passing of development.

More frequent, however, for preschool children (and also in many adults!) is to be afraid of the toilet and therefore refuses to pee and poop there. What can parents do to face this seemingly inexplicable fear?

First of all, it is important to understand that it is not so obvious for a child to immediately achieve good sphincter control: this developmental phase is complex and requires many resources. Children may fear falling into the toilet or being sucked into it in some way, so they struggle to evacuate safely.

To tackle this problem, we must certainly not ignore this signal.

As I have repeated several times in this book, it is always advisable to convey naturalness when in the bathroom, involving the child in various tasks and making her familiar with it, creating a kind of play and fun. For example, you could have her use the toilet brush as a "weapon" or have her flush the toilet.

You can also take dolls or puppets to the bathroom so that she feels reassured. You could also personify the toilet by greeting it; this would create greater confidence with the object.

You must always avoid, when the child poops, to use words like "that stinks" and "that disgusting", children do not want to feel stinky and above all they do not want to do something that disgusts their mother. So, when the baby evacuates, you have to praise her and tell her that she was a good girl and her mother is very proud of her.

Problems and Solutions

Understanding if you need to take your baby's diaper off is never very easy. There are parents who are based on age, but in reality, the best thing to do would be to rely on certain cues your child gives you every day.

Not noticing whether the baby is ready or not

You need to have good ability to observe the signals and not get anxious about having to eliminate the diaper, perhaps on the advice of the pediatrician or some friend.

Some may recommend that you continue the process once it has begun while others may recommend that you have the diaper put on again if your baby is still not quite ready.

If the child suddenly finds herself having to perform a task for which she does not feel ready yet, anxieties and fears could easily emerge. These would lead the child to even refuse to do her needs for hours (frequent is the case of children who become constipated precisely because they experienced the transition to the potty as a stretch).

In addition to this, a study in the early 1950s highlighted how, in the transition phase to the use of the toilet, not only the maturity reached, but also the temperament of the child, which the authors divide into 3 categories: easy, slow to warm up and lively / difficult.

While the easy child adapts quickly and without much difficulty to the changes, the slow-warming child will need slower rhythms and more reserved situations to reach her goal. The lively / difficult child will have a lot of difficulty adapting to the demands of the environment, will be irritable and more unpredictable, especially in the rhythm and signaling of her needs.

I advise you, always as far as possible, according to your availability of time and desire, to wait for everyone to be ready for the process. As a result, everything will be simpler and more harmonious.

Do not communicate with the baby

One can make the mistake, often due to too much haste, of not preparing the child calmly and in time, for example by providing her with books to consult or by telling her stories.

In the transition period from diaper to toilet, you can start by presenting the potty as a game and not an imposition or a challenge to be overcome in the shortest possible time. Keep in mind that the baby does not know why she has to do it, since the diaper has been one of her most faithful companions since she was born: she has the right to know why she has to change.

Once you have entered the topic, you will move on to practice. It will be a pleasant and fun time to choose the potty or the reducer with the favorite shapes or colors of the child and maybe it would be better to do some tests with water first or with a doll with which you can simulate the use of the reducer.

In addition, sitting on the toilet and showing how to use it will be an excellent incentive to use the reducer.

Sudden events that cause regression

Events such as a parent's business trip, or the birth of a sibling, or a change of home can all be reasons that could lead the child to wet the bed again at night.

However, this shouldn't make you more alarmed than expected as even up to 5 years of age it is normal to pee in bed.

Always treat it very calmly and don't make the child feel wrong.

Better not to wait for the entrance to kindergarten

When it comes to determining what is the best time to start the transition to the toilet, many families passively let external events determine it such as entry to kindergarten, where teachers are not required to change diapers, or in the vicinity of particular events, such as trips or moves or the return to work of one or both parents.

Yet, the moment in which you will have to switch to underwear is a passage that will at some point mark each individual life. It is advisable to set up your daily actions and habits so that you become familiar with the potty or the toilet right away.

As we said before, children can get used to sitting on the toilet or on the reducer since they are able to stand by themselves in this position. It does not matter where: the child is more independently on the potty, while the toilet with the reducer is a rather complex destination to climb and always requires the help of an adult.

Or, when possible, you can also try to set up a toilet routine. Therefore, you can associate the use of the toilet at particular times of the day: as soon as you wake up, before going out or going to bed, in the middle of the morning and after an afternoon nap.

Parental Behavior

For parents and especially for mothers, this phase can be very stressful and can jeopardize the harmony of the home environment.

Sometimes it is possible to become filled with doubts that can cause frustration. It is normal to think that the correct actions are not being done or that you have not waited long enough etc. Things get more difficult if the baby is unmanageable due to the fact that she is complaining or crying. This leads you to be more nervous and will create a kind of vicious circle.

Another thing, however, is to observe the signals in the child that make you understand that she is potentially ready, but not wanting to follow them.

Perhaps you are not motivated enough or due to lack of time for work or other, the start of the phase is postponed. However, this will result as a lack of listening in the child who will continue to rely on the diaper and will have to relearn again to understand her own stimuli and to control them (probably with greater difficulty).

Furthermore, I advise you, if you undertake this phase, to do it in the most consistent and disciplined way possible.

For example, answering the child who suddenly asks us to pee when you are in the city center "Love, this time do it in the diaper" would be an attitude that can generate confusion in your child, who will not be able to distinguish when to pee herself off and when in the potty. If, on the other hand, despite the possibility that she does it in the diaper due to the distance from the bathrooms, inviting her to pee by removing the diaper will communicate to your child that you listen to her needs. This will help her to learn to control herself and stimulates her cause she will know that, as soon as possible, you will enable her to free herself.

You may think that children are not ready, but most of the time the parents are not ready to lead their children towards the big leap.

If you remain calm and in control, if you accept that like any path this too is marked by progressions and regressions, no one will get hurt. Indeed, family life will be enriched with nice anecdotes to tell during family reunions.

Outdoor "Emergencies"

In the early stages of the transition between the diaper and the potty, as we said earlier, absorbent panties will be a good help. When you are away from home and the baby is unable to pee in time, she will not dirty her clothes and she will not feel uncomfortable.

If you really can't find a public toilet, or if that isn't right for you, you can choose the quickest way, find a small plant or an isolated area in which to have your child empty her bladder. Let the boy or girl understand that this is an emergency solution, not a habit. But be careful because in some cities this "practice" is prohibited by the law and you may incur a fine.

Some parents choose to carry a potty in the car so it can be pulled out whenever needed. This is especially useful if you are traveling long distances.

There are some very interesting potty models. Some are space-saving, they fold and become flat, can be slipped into a bag or stored in the lower compartment of the stroller. They are versatile because they act as a potty with the fins mounted vertically or as a reducer with the fins arranged horizontally. They are not expensive, they are hygienic because pee and poo are collected in the supplied bags that fold in a few moments and are thrown away without leaving unpleasant odors.

Here are other suggestions to limit emergencies as much as possible:

Try to leave the house only after the baby has just used the bathroom. This will limit the need to run to the bathroom with a half-full shopping cart

The use of panties for potty training will allow the child to feel comfortable at home as well as traveling

Find out the location of the nearest toilets, wherever you go. Take a quick tour to check the status before she needs it, so that she feels comfortable when she feels the urge to use the toilet

Bring a change of clothes with you as they may always come in handy

If you are almost at the finish line of toilet training and your child is no longer wearing potty training panties, disposable sheets can act as a comfortable cover for the car seat in case of minor accidents

Public Restrooms

It's very normal for newly trained (or still-learning) children not to want to go potty in public restrooms, which appear to be unfamiliar, daunting and noisy.

One easy solution: use the toilet before you leave the house. Reduce your trips to a minimum and keep your trips quick and convenient when you go out so that, when the urge pops up again, you'll be home in time to go potty in a familiar location.

The biggest problem with public toilets is undoubtedly noise. This can be very disturbing for sensitive children.

You can reduce the noise by:

- Bringing earmuffs or headphones of children's size with you

- Avoiding toilets with plenty of doors. If there's one, look for a family restroom; this is usually a smaller space with only a toilet and sink, much like your home bathroom

- Covering the sensor on an automatic flush toilet so that it won't annoy your kids. You can use a sticky piece of paper or your hand

- Letting your child go and wait by the sink while you're flushing

- Carrying your hand towels or paper towels, so you don't have to use hand dryers

Remember to always strictly follow the sanitary rules when you are in a public bathroom.

It is also important to teach the child not to touch "everything" in public toilet. If they are old enough to stand on their own legs, this is doable, but if they are small, the game can be more difficult.

Also, children tend to hold onto the toilet seat quite automatically and, not knowing who has been in that bathroom, they could really risk getting sick (as children tend to put their fingers in their mouths). Eventually you can clean the toilet, but it is difficult to carry cleaning products around, especially during an emergency (and let's be honest, who would like to clean a toilet in a public bathroom?).

Another possibility is travel covers, which are very comfortable because they are plasticized and very wide, fantastic for those who take long trips with their children.

At the moment of use, just open them, place them on the board. When the child finishes her business, you can throw them away. Some models are equipped with adhesive strips so there is no danger of them moving. They are disposable, they are waterproof and can be found in any supermarket. They are also easier to use than toilet paper on the edge of the toilet. The toilet paper is not so hygienic for this purpose because placing it on the toilet, it could still get wet due to residues left by someone else.

Emergency Kit

Now I will list some of the items you can take with you when you are away from home:

- wet wipes
- anti-mosquito wipes, especially for the summer
- toilet paper wipes, which refresh and are biodegradable
- plasticized toilet seats
- small towel, as it may be needed to clean the baby
- patches of various sizes
- anti-redness cream

- panties
- plastic bag, for storing dirty or wet wipes or towels
- markers and paper, to entertain her especially when she is in public places and there are no children to play with.

Conclusion

There are many ways to potty train. Whatever method you use, stock up on underwear and work hard to stay positive, or at least push through it with a smile, because they're watching you. Parents, you are one of the most important figures for your children because they will take an example from you.

Ensure you use the evening to "charge the batteries" whatever way you prefer and, most of all, acknowledge that using the toilet is a big life skill and you are in this together.

Be cool, calm, and confident, and your child will follow your lead. You'll be so proud of your kid (and yourself!) when you're done.

So, I hope you will treasure my advice and wish you the best of luck!

www.ingramcontent.com/pod-product-compliance
Lightning Source LLC
Chambersburg PA
CBHW030447220526
45464CB00006B/2443